The Complete Keto Diet for Beginners

2020-2021

Effortless Recipes to Lose Weight and Reverse Disease

(How I Dropped 30 Pounds in 30-Day)

Dr Casser Scott

Table of Contents

Introduction

As you probably know, losing weight is not that easy.

If you're like most people who have tried many different weight loss programs, you'll find that it's not difficult to get positive results in the beginning.

After a couple of weeks, you'd start to drop a few pounds, and you'd be happy about it.

But the real challenge lies in keeping the weight off.

This is why, many experts suggest getting into a weight loss program that can become a lifestyle for you.

This way, you can achieve your ideal weight and maintain it for a long time.

One example of such weight loss program is the ketogenic diet.

Also known as the keto diet, this one can eventually become a lifestyle for you if you are able to do it right.

And this does not only keep the pounds off, it also improves your overall health.

Are you ready to get to know more about this amazing diet program?

Then let's get started.

Chapter 1: Overview

What is Keto Diet?

The keto diet is a diet program that restricts carbohydrate intake among its users. But that's not all. It's not your average low-carb diet. What makes this one different is that it encourages intake of fat (particularly good fats) and requires adequate intake of protein.

How Does the Keto Diet Work?

Just like anyone who's starting out with the keto diet, you are probably asking this same question: how can you lose weight if you are going to take in more fats?

To understand how the keto diet works, one must know about how the body's metabolic processes work.

When the body takes in both carbs and fats, it prioritizes the use of carb as fuel for energy. It burns carb and uses it to energize the body. What about the fats? The body doesn't have much use for it so it stores the fat in your tissues, and this is what causes weight gain.

Now if you don't take in any carbs but take in more fats, the body is forced to enter a state called "ketosis".

This is a state in which the body burns the fats stored in your body, and the fats you're consuming in order to get the energy it needs to function properly. And this is what causes weight loss.

It's not that difficult to understand why the keto diet is effective if you know exactly how your body works.

Foods You Can Eat

As with most diet programs, there's a list of foods you can eat and cannot eat in the ketogenic diet.

Here's a list of foods that you should include in your diet:

- Meat – Beef, pork, lamb, steak, ham, sausage, bacon
- Poultry – Chicken, turkey, duck
- Seafood – Fatty fish such as salmon, tuna, trout, and other seafood like shrimp, crabs, crabmeat, seashells

- Eggs – Preferably omega 3 eggs
- Dairy products – Butter, cream, milk, cheese (cheddar, Parmesan cheese, cream cheese, blue cheese, mozzarella cheese and so on)
- Nuts and seeds – Almonds, flax seeds, chia seeds, walnuts, pistachios
- Healthy cooking oils – Avocado oil, olive oil, coconut oil
- Avocados
- Low-carb vegetables – Leafy greens, onion, garlic, tomatoes, bell peppers, sweet peppers, peppers
- Condiments – Salt, pepper, herbs and spices
- Keto products – Keto bread, keto crackers, keto sweetener and so on

Foods You Cannot Eat

As for those that you cannot eat while on this diet, you have to avoid foods that are high in carbohydrates and sugar. It's imperative to steer clear of grains, starches and sugary beverages among others.

Here's a list for you to remind you of what's off limits:

- Food and drinks high in sugar – Soda, fruit juices, cakes, pastries, candies
- Grains and starches – White rice, white pasta, cereal
- Fruits except for avocados, dried fruits and berries
- Beams and legumes
- Condiments and sauces high in fat and sugar
- Alcoholic beverages

Steps to Get Started

To make sure that you are on the right path right from the beginning, here are the proper steps to follow as you embark on your ketogenic diet.

Step # 1 – Do your homework

Of course, the first step is to do ample research about the keto diet. It's not enough that you know what it is and how it works. You need to know the proper steps in following this diet.

The proper keto diet is composed of 70 percent fat, 20 percent protein and 10 percent fat. This means that if you are on a 2,000-calorie diet, you will need to take in about 160 grams of fat, about 40 grams of carbs and about 70 grams of protein.

Step # 2 – Consult your doctor

Before getting started with this diet or any other diet program, you need to consult your doctor first.

Why? Some diet programs are not advisable for some groups of people.

It's a must that you are in good health condition before starting this diet, which is why you need to go for a checkup with your doctor.

Aside from pregnant and nursing mothers, the keto diet is also not suitable for people who have existing heart disease or are at risk of heart conditions, and who have type 1 diabetes, pancreas or liver condition.

Step # 3 – Consult a dietician

Next, you should also consult a professional nutritionist or dietician to help formulate a diet program that will work for you.

You can also get into the keto diet on your own with proper research and with the help of this book, but of course, it's also a great idea if you get professional help.

Step # 4 – Make a plan

It's now time for you to make your own plan.

First, you need to make a weekly menu or if you can, a 30-day menu plan. After the recipes section of this book, you will find a sample 30-day menu plan that you can follow.

Next, list down the ingredients that you will need for the menu that you plan to prepare for yourself. The purpose of this is for you to save time and energy during food preparation, to ensure that everything you need is ready before you start working in the kitchen.

Step # 5 – Make gradual changes in your diet

This is a crucial step for anyone who's starting out on the keto diet.

Don't make drastic changes in your diet as this might overwhelm you and cause you to backslide halfway through the diet.

Make small steps as you make your way through the keto diet program.

For example, eliminate carbs slowly. You can start by avoiding bread but you can still eat rice or pasta. Then as days go by, you can start to eliminate rice and pasta as well.

This gives your body ample time to adjust to your new diet.

Tips for Cooking at Home

Here are the tips for success to keep in mind when it comes to cooking at home while on a keto diet:

- Get rid of temptations – Do not stock rice, pasta and other food or ingredients that are high in carb and sugar.
- Make a menu plan and list down the ingredients that you'll need – This will guide you during grocery shopping to save you time and effort.
- Go for pre-cut or pre-prepared ingredients – Another way to save time and energy is to go for ingredients that have already been pre-prepared. For example, if you need pesto, you can buy prepared pesto in the grocery. Just check the label to ensure that it fits your diet program.
- Make meals in advance – You might also want to prepare dishes in advance and freeze later for quick and convenient reheating. There are many dishes that are ideal for freezing that you can check out.

Tips for Eating Out

Eating out can be a challenge when you're in the keto diet. Here are some tips that can definitely help:

- Check the menu in advance – Most restaurants now have websites that contain their menu, or at least their house specialties that you can check out in advance to see if the selections are suitable for your diet. If not, you can skip this restaurant and find another one.
- Inquire for alternatives – If you've been invited by a friend or family member to eat out, you can inquire with the server if they have alternatives that they can serve you with. For example, they might have zucchini noodles for their pasta offerings.
- Avoid eating out – If you are just getting stressed out with eating out, then you might as well just stay at home and prepare your own food. The convenience of eating out is defeated when you get all stressed out worrying about your diet.

So, there you go, all the things you need to know to get started with the keto diet.

Let's now proceed to the fun part: cooking keto-friendly recipes!

Chapter 2: Breakfast Recipes

Cheesy Omelet with Bacon & Black Beans

Preparation Time: 20 minutes
Cooking Time: 20 minutes
Servings: 6

Ingredients:

- 8 eggs
- ½ cup milk
- Salt and pepper to taste
- Cooking spray
- ¾ cup black beans, rinsed and drained
- 1 cup crispy bacon bits
- 1 cup red bell pepper, chopped
- 6 tablespoons Monterey Jack cheese, shredded

Method:

1. Preheat your oven to 325 degrees F.
2. In a bowl, beat the eggs.
3. Pour in milk and season with salt and pepper.
4. Spray your muffin pan with oil.
5. Divide the beans, bacon and bell pepper among the cups.
6. Pour the egg mixture on top.
7. Top with the cheese.
8. Bake for 20 minutes.

Nutritional Value:

- Calories 187
- Total Fat 18.8 g
- Saturated Fat 7 g
- Cholesterol 355 mg
- Sodium 361 mg
- Total Carbohydrate 8.4 g
- Dietary Fiber 2.7 g
- Protein 12.9 g
- Total Sugars 3 g
- Potassium 291 mg

Omelet with Sun-Dried Tomatoes & Sausage

Preparation Time: 20 minutes
Cooking Time: 20 minutes
Servings: 6

Ingredients:

- 8 eggs
- ½ cup milk
- Salt and pepper to taste
- Cooking spray
- 1 cup roasted red peppers, chopped
- 1 cup sausage, cooked and crumbled
- 6 tablespoons mozzarella cheese, shredded
- ¼ cup sun-dried tomatoes, chopped

Method:

1. Preheat your oven to 325 degrees F.
2. In a bowl, beat the eggs and milk.
3. Sprinkle with salt and pepper.
4. Spray your muffin cup with oil.
5. Add the red peppers and sausage to the muffin cups.
6. Pour egg mixture on top.
7. Add cheese on top of egg mixture.
8. Bake for 20 minutes.

Nutritional Value:

- Calories 197
- Total Fat 19.1 g
- Saturated Fat 8 g
- Cholesterol 254 mg
- Sodium 462 mg
- Total Carbohydrate 6 g
- Dietary Fiber 0.8 g
- Protein 12.3 g
- Total Sugars 4 g
- Potassium 272 mg

Chaffle Sandwich with Bacon & Avocado

Preparation Time: 15 minutes
Cooking Time: 5 minutes
Servings: 8

Ingredients:

- 10 eggs
- 2 slices bacon, cooked crispy and chopped
- 1 ½ cups cheddar cheese, shredded
- Pepper to taste
- Cooking spray
- 2 tomatoes, sliced
- 2 avocado, diced
- 4 lettuce leaves, torn

Method:

1. In a bowl, beat the eggs.
2. Add the bacon and cheese.
3. Season with pepper.
4. Spray your waffle iron with oil.
5. Pour the mixture into the iron.
6. Cook for 5 minutes.
7. Top with the tomato, avocado and lettuce.

Nutritional Value:

- Calories 259
- Total Fat 20 g
- Saturated Fat 6.6 g
- Cholesterol 252 mg
- Sodium 244 mg
- Total Carbohydrate 6.8 g
- Dietary Fiber 3.8 g
- Protein 14 g
- Total Sugars 2 g
- Potassium 446 mg

Bacon, Mushroom & Spinach Quiches

Preparation Time: 20 minutes
Cooking Time: 45 minutes
Servings: 6

Ingredients:

- 2 tablespoons olive oil
- 4 oz. oyster mushrooms
- 4 oz. shiitake mushrooms
- 1 cup onion, sliced thinly
- 1 tablespoon garlic, minced
- 2 teaspoons fresh thyme, minced
- 5 oz. spinach, chopped
- 8 eggs, beaten
- ¼ cup milk
- 1 cup Gruyère cheese, shredded
- Salt and pepper to taste
- 2 teaspoons Dijon mustard

Method:

1. Preheat your oven to 325 degrees F.
2. In a pan over medium heat, pour oil and cook mushrooms for 4 to 5 minutes.
3. Stir and cook for another 5 minutes.
4. Put the onion and garlic in the pan. Cook for 3 minutes.
5. Stir in spinach and cook for 2 minutes.
6. Combine the remaining ingredients in a bowl.
7. Add mushroom mixture.
8. Pour into a greased muffin pan.
9. Bake for 30 minutes.

Nutritional Value:

- Calories 236
- Total Fat 16.4 g
- Saturated Fat 5.8 g
- Cholesterol 266 mg
- Sodium 459 mg

- Total Carbohydrate 7.1 g
- Dietary Fiber 1.5 g
- Protein 15.5 g
- Total Sugars 4 g
- Potassium 443 mg

Greek Omelet with Feta

Preparation Time: 20 minutes
Cooking Time: 35 minutes
Servings: 6

Ingredients:

- Cooking spray
- 2 tablespoons olive oil
- 1 yellow onion, chopped
- 1 tablespoon oregano, chopped
- 1 red bell pepper, chopped
- Salt and pepper to taste
- 8 large eggs, beaten
- ½ cup milk
- 1 cup feta cheese, crumbled
- 2 cups spinach, chopped
- ¼ cup Kalamata olives, sliced

Method:

1. Preheat your oven to 325 degrees F.
2. Spray your muffin pan with oil.
3. Pour oil into a pan over medium heat.
4. Cook onion, oregano and bell pepper for 5 minutes.
5. In a bowl, mix the remaining ingredients along with the onion mixture.
6. Sprinkle with salt and pepper.
7. Pour into muffin cups.
8. Bake for 30 minutes.

Nutritional Value:

- Calories 226
- Total Fat 16.7 g
- Saturated Fat 5.8 g
- Cholesterol 266 mg
- Sodium 466 mg
- Total Carbohydrate 6.7 g
- Dietary Fiber 1.3 g
- Protein 12.7 g
- Total Sugars 4 g
- Potassium 211 mg

Cheesy Spinach & Broccoli Omelet

Preparation Time: 15 minutes
Cooking Time: 10 minutes
Serving: 1

Ingredients:

- 2 teaspoons olive oil
- ¼ cup spinach, chopped
- ¼ cup broccoli, chopped
- 1 egg, beaten
- 2 tablespoons cheddar cheese, shredded
- 1 tablespoon milk
- Salt to taste
- 1 tablespoon sour cream
- Chopped chives

Method:

1. Add oil to a pan over medium heat.
2. Cook spinach and broccoli for 5 minutes.
3. In a bowl, mix the egg, cheese and milk.
4. Pour into the pan.
5. Mix to combine.
6. Season with salt.
7. Cook for 2 minutes.
8. Serve with sour cream and garnish with chives.

Nutritional Value:

- Calories 244
- Total Fat 20.6 g
- Saturated Fat 7 g
- Cholesterol 206 mg
- Sodium 478 mg
- Total Carbohydrate 3.1 g
- Dietary Fiber 0.6 g
- Protein 11.5 g
- Total Sugars 1 g
- Potassium X mg

Toast with Raspberries & Mascarpone

Preparation Time: 5 minutes
Cooking Time: 0 minutes
Serving: 1

Ingredients:

- 2 tablespoons mascarpone cheese
- 1 slice keto bread, toasted
- ¼ cup raspberries, chopped
- Mint leaves

Method:

1. Spread cheese on top of the keto bread.
2. Top with the raspberries and mint leaves.

Nutritional Value:

- Calories 326
- Total Fat 27.3 g
- Saturated Fat 14.2 g
- Cholesterol 70 mg
- Sodium 130 mg
- Total Carbohydrate 5 g
- Dietary Fiber 4.1 g
- Protein 7.9 g
- Total Sugars 3 g
- Potassium 115 mg

Omelet with Herbs & Goat Cheese

Preparation Time: 10 minutes
Cooking Time: 5 minutes
Servings: 2

Ingredients:

- 4 eggs, beaten
- ½ cup goat cheese, crumbled
- 2 tablespoons milk
- Salt and pepper to taste
- 1 tablespoon olive oil
- Chopped parsley
- Chopped chives

Method:

1. Beat the eggs in a bowl.
2. Add the goat cheese, milk, salt and pepper.
3. Pour oil into a pan over medium heat.
4. Add the egg mixture to the pan.
5. Sprinkle with the parsley and chives.
6. Cook for 5 minutes.

Nutritional Value:

- Calories 227
- Total Fat 16.9 g
- Saturated Fat 6.7 g
- Cholesterol 397 mg
- Sodium 386 mg
- Total Carbohydrate 2.5 g
- Dietary Fiber 0.9 g
- Protein 16.6 g
- Total Sugars 1 g
- Potassium 183 mg

Omelet with Arugula & Tomatoes

Preparation Time: 15 minutes
Cooking Time: 5 minutes
Servings: 4

Ingredients:

- Cooking spray
- 8 eggs, beaten
- Salt and pepper to taste
- 1 cup arugula, sliced
- 1 cup tomato, chopped
- ½ cup feta cheese, crumbled
- ¼ cup Kalamata olives, pitted and sliced

Method:

1. Spray your pan with oil.
2. In a bowl, beat the eggs and season with salt and pepper.
3. Put the pan over medium heat.
4. Cook the egg mixture for 1 minute, stirring.
5. Add the rest of the ingredients on top.
6. Fold and flip.
7. Cook for 1 minute.

Nutritional Value:

- Calories 118
- Total Fat 13.5 g
- Saturated Fat 5 g
- Cholesterol 25 mg
- Sodium 562 mg
- Total Carbohydrate 5 g
- Dietary Fiber 1.3 g
- Protein 16 g
- Total Sugars 2 g
- Potassium 296 mg

Keto Toast with Chicken & Cucumber

Preparation Time: 5 minutes
Cooking Time: 0 minutes
Serving: 1

Ingredients:

- 1 slice keto bread, toasted
- 2 tablespoons cucumber, chopped
- ¼ cup cooked chicken, shredded
- Chopped cilantro
- Salt to taste

Method:

1. Top the keto bread with chicken, cucumber and cilantro.
2. Sprinkle with salt.

Nutritional Value:

- Calories 141
- Total Fat 16 g
- Saturated Fat 6 g
- Cholesterol 30 mg
- Sodium 300 mg
- Total Carbohydrate 3 g
- Dietary Fiber 2 g
- Protein 7.6 g
- Total Sugars 2 g
- Potassium 174 mg

Chapter 3: Beef Recipes

Beef-Stuffed Mushrooms

Preparation Time: 20 minutes
Cooking Time: 25 minutes
Servings: 4

Ingredients:

- 4 mushrooms, stemmed
- 3 tablespoons olive oil, divided
- 1 yellow onion, sliced thinly
- 1 red bell pepper, sliced into strips
- 1 green bell pepper, sliced into strips
- Salt and pepper to taste
- 8 oz. beef, sliced thinly
- 3 oz. provolone cheese, sliced
- Chopped parsley

Method:

1. Preheat your oven to 350 degrees F.
2. Arrange the mushrooms on a baking pan.
3. Brush with oil.
4. Add the remaining oil to a pan over medium heat.
5. Cook onion and bell peppers for 5 minutes.
6. Season with salt and pepper.
7. Place onion mixture on a plate.
8. Cook the beef in the pan for 5 minutes.
9. Sprinkle with salt and pepper.
10. Add the onion mixture back to the pan.
11. Mix well.
12. Fill the mushrooms with the beef mixture and cheese.
13. Bake in the oven for 15 minutes.

Nutritional Value:

- Calories 333
- Total Fat 20.3 g

- Saturated Fat 6.7 g
- Cholesterol 61 mg
- Sodium 378 mg
- Total Carbohydrate 8.2 g
- Dietary Fiber 3.7 g
- Protein 25.2 g
- Total Sugars 7 g
- Potassium 789 mg

Grilled Steak with Tomato Salad

Preparation Time: 15 minutes
Cooking Time: 10 minutes
Servings: 4

Ingredients:

- 2 teaspoons garlic, minced
- 4 cups tomatoes, sliced
- ½ cup cilantro, chopped
- ¼ cup olive oil
- Salt and pepper to taste
- 1 lb. flank steak

Method:

1. Preheat your grill.
2. In a bowl, toss garlic, tomatoes and cilantro in olive oil. Set aside.
3. Sprinkle steak with salt and pepper.
4. Grill the steak for 4 minutes per side.
5. Transfer to a cutting board.
6. Let cool and then slice.
7. Serve the steak with the tomato salad.

Nutritional Value:

- Calories 346
- Total Fat 25.1 g
- Saturated Fat 5 g
- Cholesterol 70 mg
- Sodium 358 mg
- Total Carbohydrate 3.9 g
- Dietary Fiber 1.1 g
- Protein 25 g
- Total Sugars 2 g
- Potassium 591 mg

Sweet & Spicy Flank Steak

Preparation Time: 20 minutes
Cooking Time: 15 minutes
Servings: 4

Ingredients:

- Salt and pepper to taste
- 1 teaspoon brown sugar
- 1 lb. flank steak
- 1 lb. bell peppers
- 1 tablespoon olive oil
- 1 teaspoon rice vinegar
- Chopped scallions

Method:

1. Preheat your broiler.
2. Mix salt, pepper and brown sugar in a bowl.
3. Season steak with this mixture.
4. In another bowl, toss bell peppers in oil.
5. Place the steak in a baking pan surrounded with bell peppers.
6. Broil for 15 minutes, flipping once.
7. Combine the remaining ingredients in a bowl.
8. Toss the roasted bell peppers in the mixture.
9. Serve steak with bell peppers.

Nutritional Value:

- Calories 263
- Total Fat 17.8 g
- Saturated Fat 7.9 g
- Cholesterol 68 mg
- Sodium 441 mg
- Total Carbohydrate 5 g
- Dietary Fiber 2.7 g
- Protein 24.6 g
- Total Sugars 8 g
- Potassium 545 mg

Rib Roast

Preparation Time: 15 minutes
Cooking Time: 3 hours
Servings: 8

Ingredients:

- 1 rib roast
- Salt to taste
- 12 cloves garlic, chopped
- 2 teaspoons lemon zest
- 6 tablespoons fresh rosemary, chopped
- 5 sprigs thyme

Method:

1. Preheat your oven to 325 degrees F.
2. Season all sides of rib roast with salt.
3. Place the rib roast in a baking pan.
4. Sprinkle with garlic, lemon zest and rosemary.
5. Add herb sprigs on top.
6. Roast for 3 hours.
7. Let rest for a few minutes and then slice and serve.

Nutritional Value:

- Calories 329
- Total Fat 27 g
- Saturated Fat 9 g
- Cholesterol 59 mg
- Sodium 498 mg
- Total Carbohydrate 5.3 g
- Dietary Fiber 1.8 g
- Protein 18 g
- Total Sugars 2 g
- Potassium 493 mg

Meatloaf with Sausage

Preparation Time: 30 minutes
Cooking Time: 50 minutes
Servings: 10

Ingredients:

- 2 tablespoons olive oil
- 1 yellow onion, chopped
- 6 cloves garlic, minced
- 1 cup celery, chopped
- 1 cup whole-wheat breadcrumbs
- 2 eggs, beaten
- ½ cup fresh parsley, chopped
- 6 tablespoons ketchup
- 1 lb. lean ground beef
- 8 oz. ground pork
- 12 oz. ground turkey
- 8 oz. sausage, removed from casing and crumbled
- 2 tablespoons Worcestershire sauce
- Salt and pepper to taste

Method:

1. Preheat your oven to 350 degrees F.
2. Spray your loaf pan with oil.
3. Pour oil into a pan over medium heat.
4. Cook onion, garlic and celery for 10 minutes.
5. Transfer onion mixture to a baking pan.
6. Stir in the rest of the ingredients.
7. Press mixture into a loaf pan.
8. Bake for 40 minutes.

Nutritional Value:

- Calories 305
- Total Fat 15.6 g
- Saturated Fat 4.6 g
- Cholesterol 119 mg

- Sodium 505 mg
- Total Carbohydrate 14.8 g
- Dietary Fiber 1.5 g
- Protein 26.7 g
- Total Sugars 6 g
- Potassium 399 mg

Beef Bourguignon

Preparation Time: 30 minutes
Cooking Time: 1 hour
Servings: 8

Ingredients:

- 2 lb. beet stew meat, sliced into cubes
- Salt and pepper to taste
- 3 tablespoons olive oil
- ¼ cup dry red wine
- 1 onion, chopped
- 4 cloves garlic, minced
- 1 cup carrot, chopped
- 1 teaspoon dried thyme
- 15 oz. canned diced tomatoes
- 1 cup beef broth
- 1 bay leaf
- 5 cups mushrooms
- 2 tablespoons cornstarch mixed with 2 tablespoons water

Method:

1. Season beef with salt and pepper.
2. Pour oil into a pan over medium heat.
3. Cook the beef for 5 minutes.
4. Pour in the wine.
5. Cook for 2 minutes.
6. Transfer to a plate and set aside.
7. Cook onion, garlic and carrots in the same pan for 5 minutes.
8. Transfer beef and onion mixture to a pressure cooker.
9. Stir in the rest of the ingredients except cornstarch mixture.
10. Seal the pot.
11. Cook on high for 40 minutes.
12. Release pressure naturally.
13. Transfer beef and veggies to a serving plate.
14. Transfer cooking liquid to a pan.
15. Stir in cornstarch mixture.

16. Simmer sauce until thickened.
17. Serve beef and veggies poured with sauce.

Nutritional Value:

- Calories 252
- Total Fat 20 g
- Saturated Fat 9 g
- Cholesterol 85 mg
- Sodium 357 mg
- Total Carbohydrate 8 g
- Dietary Fiber 2.4 g
- Protein 24 g
- Total Sugars 7 g
- Potassium 905 mg

Prime Rib

Preparation Time: 20 minutes
Cooking Time: 3 hours
Servings: 14

Ingredients:

- 4 cloves garlic, chopped
- Salt and pepper to taste
- 1 teaspoon fresh rosemary, chopped
- 1 tablespoon fresh thyme, chopped
- 3 tablespoons olive oil
- 1 rib roast

Method:

1. Crush the garlic and sprinkle with salt.
2. Stir in the herbs, pepper and oil.
3. Form a paste from the mixture.
4. Rub the mixture all over the rib roast.
5. Roast in the oven at 275 degrees F for 3 hours.

Nutritional Value:

- Calories 459
- Total Fat 36.9 g
- Saturated Fat 14.4 g
- Cholesterol 101 mg
- Sodium 488 mg
- Total Carbohydrate 0.5 g
- Dietary Fiber 0.1 g
- Protein 29.4 g
- Total Sugars 2 g
- Potassium 411 mg

Seared Steak

Preparation Time: 15 minutes
Cooking Time: 10 minutes
Servings: 4

Ingredients:

- 1 lb. sirloin steak
- Salt and pepper to taste
- 2 tablespoons olive oil
- 4 cloves garlic, minced
- 1 sprig fresh rosemary
- 3 sprigs fresh sage
- 5 sprigs fresh thyme
- 1 lb. escarole, chopped

Method:

1. Season both sides of steak with salt and pepper.
2. Pour oil into a pan over medium heat.
3. Cook steak for 3 minutes.
4. Add the garlic and herbs.
5. Cook for 5 minutes.
6. Top the steak with herbs and garlic.

Nutritional Value:

- Calories 244
- Total Fat 11.8 g
- Saturated Fat 2.5 g
- Cholesterol 59 mg
- Sodium 394 mg
- Total Carbohydrate 8 g
- Dietary Fiber 8.2 g
- Protein 25.5 g
- Total Sugars 1 g
- Potassium 1111 mg

Steak Salad

Preparation Time: 30 minutes
Cooking Time: 10 minutes
Servings: 4

Ingredients:

- ½ teaspoon red pepper flakes
- ½ teaspoon paprika
- 1 teaspoon ground cumin
- Salt and pepper to taste
- 1 pound flank steak
- 3 tablespoons olive oil
- 1 onion, chopped
- 1 clove garlic, grated
- ½ teaspoon whole-grain mustard
- 2 tablespoons red-wine vinegar
- 1 teaspoon lemon zest
- 1 tablespoon lemon juice
- 1 cup Greek yogurt
- 4 cups Romaine lettuce, sliced
- 1 cucumber, diced
- 1 cup tomatoes, chopped
- Chopped chives
- Chopped mint leaves

Method:

1. Preheat your grill.
2. Mix red pepper flakes, paprika, cumin, salt and pepper.
3. Season steak with this mixture.
4. Grill steak for 4 to 5 minutes per side.
5. Transfer to a cutting board.
6. Let rest and then slice into strips.
7. Combine olive oil, onion, garlic, mustard, vinegar, lemon zest, lemon juice and yogurt in a bowl. Set aside.
8. Arrange the lettuce on a serving platter.
9. Top with the steak, cucumber and tomatoes.

10. Sprinkle with chopped herbs.
11. Serve steak salad with dressing.

Nutritional Value:

- Calories 381
- Total Fat 21.2 g
- Saturated Fat 9 g
- Cholesterol 76 mg
- Sodium 594 mg
- Total Carbohydrate 4.9 g
- Dietary Fiber 5 g
- Protein 33.4 g
- Total Sugars 8 g
- Potassium 1114 mg

Beef Stir Fry

Preparation Time: 15 minutes
Cooking Time: 10 minutes
Servings: 4

Ingredients:

- 1 tablespoon soy sauce
- 1 tablespoon ginger, minced
- 1 teaspoon cornstarch
- 1 teaspoon dry sherry
- 12 oz. beef, sliced into strips
- 1 teaspoon toasted sesame oil
- 2 tablespoons oyster sauce
- 1 lb. baby bok choy, sliced
- 3 tablespoons chicken broth

Method:

1. Mix soy sauce, ginger, cornstarch and dry sherry in a bowl.
2. Toss the beef in the mixture.
3. Pour oil into a pan over medium heat.
4. Cook the beef for 5 minutes, stirring.
5. Add oyster sauce, bok choy and chicken broth to the pan.
6. Cook for 1 minute.

Nutritional Value:

- Calories 247
- Total Fat 15.8 g
- Saturated Fat 4 g
- Cholesterol 69 mg
- Sodium 569 mg
- Total Carbohydrate 6.3 g
- Dietary Fiber 1.1 g
- Protein 25 g
- Total Sugars 3 g
- Potassium 765 mg

Chapter 4: Pork Recipes

Grilled Pork Tenderloin

Preparation Time: 15 minutes
Cooking Time: 30 minutes
Servings: 4

Ingredients:

- 1 lb. pork tenderloin
- 2 tablespoons olive oil, divided
- Salt to taste
- ½ teaspoon chipotle chili powder
- 2 teaspoons fresh thyme, chopped
- ¼ cup shallots, chopped
- 2 cups cherries, pitted and sliced in half
- 2 tablespoons dry red wine
- 2 tablespoons fresh basil, chopped

Method:

1. Preheat your grill.
2. Brush pork with half of the oil.
3. Sprinkle with salt, chili powder and thyme.
4. Grill for 20 minutes, flipping once.
5. Transfer to a cutting board.
6. Let rest and then slice.
7. Add remaining oil to a pan over medium heat.
8. Cook shallots for 2 minutes.
9. Stir in cherries. Cook for 5 minutes.
10. Pour in wine.
11. Cook for 2 minutes.
12. Serve pork with cherries and sauce.

Nutritional Value:

- Calories 244
- Total Fat 9.6 g
- Saturated Fat 1.8 g

- Cholesterol 70 mg
- Sodium 504 mg
- Total Carbohydrate 15 g
- Dietary Fiber 1.9 g
- Protein 23.8 g
- Total Sugars 10 g
- Potassium 656 mg

Sweet & Sour Pork

Preparation Time: 15 minutes
Cooking Time: 15 minutes
Servings: 4

Ingredients:

- 1 lb. pork chops
- Salt and pepper to taste
- ½ cup sesame seeds
- 2 tablespoons peanut oil
- 2 tablespoons soy sauce
- 3 tablespoons apricot jam
- Chopped scallions

Method:

1. Season pork chops with salt and pepper.
2. Press sesame seeds on both sides of pork.
3. Pour oil into a pan over medium heat.
4. Cook pork for 3 to 5 minutes per side.
5. Transfer to a plate.
6. In a bowl, mix soy sauce and apricot jam.
7. Simmer for 3 minutes.
8. Pour sauce over the pork and garnish with scallions before serving.

Nutritional Value:

- Calories 414
- Total Fat 27.5 g
- Saturated Fat 5.6 g
- Cholesterol 68 mg
- Sodium 607 mg
- Total Carbohydrate 12.9 g
- Dietary Fiber 1.8 g
- Protein 29 g
- Total Sugars 9 g
- Potassium 332 mg

Roasted Pork Shoulder

Preparation Time: 15 minutes
Cooking Time: 2 hours and 30 minutes
Servings: 8

Ingredients:

- 2 tablespoons olive oil
- 2 tablespoons garlic, minced
- 1 tablespoon thyme, chopped
- 2 tablespoons fresh sage, chopped
- 1 tablespoon lemon zest
- 1 teaspoon ground cumin
- Salt and pepper to taste
- 4 lb. pork shoulder roast

Method:

1. Mix all ingredients except pork in a bowl.
2. Rub the mixture all over the pork roast.
3. Marinate for 1 hour.
4. Preheat your oven to 450 degrees F.
5. Place pork in a baking pan.
6. Roast for 20 to 30 minutes.
7. Lower temperature to 325 degrees F.
8. Roast for 2 hours.
9. Let rest for 5 minutes and slice.

Nutritional Value:

- Calories 254
- Total Fat 14.6 g
- Saturated Fat 4.9 g
- Cholesterol 69 mg
- Sodium 374 mg
- Total Carbohydrate 8.3 g
- Dietary Fiber 0.2 g
- Protein 18 g
- Total Sugars 6 g
- Potassium 302 mg

Pork Braised in Wine

Preparation Time: 30 minutes
Cooking Time: 2 hours and 40 minutes
Servings: 8

Ingredients:

- 2 lb. pork shoulder, sliced into cubes
- Salt and pepper to taste
- 1 tablespoon olive oil
- 1 onion, chopped
- 2 cloves garlic, chopped
- ½ cup celery, chopped
- 1 carrot, chopped
- 1 bay leaf
- 4 fresh thyme sprigs
- 2 tablespoons tomato paste
- 1 cup dry red wine
- 2 cups beef broth
- 1 cup water

Method:

1. Preheat your oven to 325 degrees F.
2. Sprinkle pork with salt and pepper.
3. Pour oil into a pan over medium heat.
4. Cook pork for 5 minutes.
5. Transfer to a plate.
6. Add onion, garlic, celery and carrot to the pan.
7. Cook for 5 minutes.
8. Stir in bay leaf and thyme.
9. Cook for 1 minute.
10. Pour in the rest of the ingredients.
11. Bring to a boil.
12. Simmer for 30 minutes.
13. Put the pork back to the pan.
14. Cover the pan with foil.
15. Place inside the oven.

16. Bake in the oven for 2 hours.
17. Shred the pork with a fork.
18. Drizzle pork with sauce and serve.

Nutritional Value:

- Calories 257
- Total Fat 14.7 g
- Saturated Fat 5 g
- Cholesterol 69 mg
- Sodium 347 mg
- Total Carbohydrate 5 g
- Dietary Fiber 1 g
- Protein 19 g
- Total Sugars 2 g
- Potassium 432 mg

Mojo Pork

Preparation Time: 15 minutes
Cooking Time: 1 hour and 10 minutes
Servings: 10

Ingredients:

- 1 pork shoulder, sliced into cubes
- 6 cloves garlic, minced
- 1 cup onion, sliced
- 3 tablespoon fresh oregano, chopped
- 2 teaspoons ground cumin
- 1 teaspoon orange zest
- 1 tablespoon orange juice
- Salt and pepper to taste
- ½ cup water
- 1 bay leaf

Method:

1. Pour oil into a pan over medium heat.
2. Cook the pork for 3 to 4 minutes per side.
3. Transfer to a bowl.
4. Add the remaining ingredients to a pressure cooker.
5. Stir in the pork.
6. Seal the pot.
7. Cook on high for 1 hour.
8. Release pressure naturally.
9. Serve pork drizzled with the sauce.

Nutritional Value:

- Calories 296
- Total Fat 19 g
- Saturated Fat 7 g
- Cholesterol 97 mg
- Sodium 444 mg
- Total Carbohydrate 4.3 g
- Dietary Fiber 0.8 g
- Protein 25 g
- Total Sugars 2 g
- Potassium 370 mg

Grilled Pork with Salsa

Preparation Time: 30 minutes
Cooking Time: 15 minutes
Servings: 4

Ingredients:

Salsa

- 1 onion, chopped
- 1 tomato, chopped
- 1 peach, chopped
- 1 apricot, chopped
- 1 tablespoon olive oil
- 1 tablespoon lime juice
- 2 tablespoons fresh cilantro, chopped
- Salt and pepper to taste

Pork

- 1 lb. pork tenderloin, sliced
- 1 tablespoon olive oil
- Salt and pepper to taste
- ½ teaspoon ground cumin
- ¾ teaspoon chili powder

Method:

1. Combine salsa ingredients in a bowl.
2. Cover and refrigerate.
3. Brush pork tenderloin with oil.
4. Season with salt, pepper, cumin and chili powder.
5. Grill pork for 5 to 7 minutes per side.
6. Slice pork and serve with salsa.

Nutritional Value:

- Calories 219
- Total Fat 9.5 g
- Saturated Fat 1.8 g

- Cholesterol 74 mg
- Sodium 512 mg
- Total Carbohydrate 8.3 g
- Dietary Fiber 1.5 g
- Protein 24 g
- Total Sugars 6 g
- Potassium 600 mg

Pork Tenderloin with Plum Chutney

Preparation Time: 20 minutes
Cooking Time: 35 minutes
Servings: 4

Ingredients:

- 1 teaspoon sesame oil
- ¼ cup onion, chopped
- 1 clove garlic, minced
- 2 plums, pitted and sliced
- 1 teaspoon grated ginger
- 1 teaspoon soy sauce
- 1 ½ teaspoons rice vinegar
- 1 teaspoon honey
- ¼ teaspoon ground coriander
- Salt to taste
- 1 lb. pork tenderloin
- Chopped scallions

Method:

1. Pour oil into a pan over medium heat.
2. Cook onion and garlic for 4 minutes.
3. Add the remaining ingredients to the pan.
4. Bring to a boil.
5. Reduce heat and simmer for 30 minutes.

Nutritional Value:

- Calories 191
- Total Fat 14 g
- Saturated Fat 9 g
- Cholesterol 74 mg
- Sodium 392 mg
- Total Carbohydrate 8 g
- Dietary Fiber 3 g
- Protein 27 g
- Total Sugars 8 g
- Potassium 1078 mg

Pork with Pears

Preparation Time: 15 minutes
Cooking Time: 40 minutes
Servings: 4

Ingredients:

- 12 oz. pork tenderloin
- Salt and pepper to taste
- 2 tablespoons onion, chopped
- 1 teaspoon fresh ginger, grated
- ¼ cup almonds, toasted and chopped
- 1 pear, chopped
- ¼ cup breadcrumbs
- ¼ cup carrot, shredded
- 1 teaspoon olive oil
- 2 tablespoons no-sugar orange jam

Method:

1. Sprinkle pork with salt and pepper.
2. Mix the rest of the ingredients except oil and orange jam.
3. Flatten the pork with meat mallet.
4. Spread pear mixture on top of the pork.
5. Roll it up.
6. Transfer to a baking pan.
7. Drizzle with oil.
8. Roast for 30 minutes.
9. Brush with orange marmalade and roast for another 10 minutes.

Nutritional Value:

- Calories 191
- Total Fat 9 g
- Saturated Fat 1 g
- Cholesterol 55 mg
- Sodium 193 mg
- Total Carbohydrate 9 g
- Dietary Fiber 2 g
- Protein 20 g
- Total Sugars 3 g
- Potassium 551 mg

Pork Taco

Preparation Time: 15 minutes
Cooking Time: 30 minutes
Servings: 4

Ingredients:

- 1 lb. pork tenderloin
- 1 teaspoon taco seasoning
- Salt to taste
- 1 onion, chopped
- 1 cup tomato, chopped
- 1 jalapeño chili pepper, chopped
- ¼ cup fresh cilantro, chopped
- 1 tablespoon lime juice
- 8 corn tortillas

Method:

1. Season pork with taco seasoning and salt.
2. Grill the pork for 30 minutes.
3. Transfer to a cutting board.
4. Slice into strips.
5. In a bowl, combine onion, tomato, chili pepper, cilantro and lime juice.
6. Top the tortillas with the pork strips and salsa.
7. Roll it up and serve.

Nutritional Value:

- Calories 238
- Total Fat 3.3 g
- Saturated Fat 0.7 g
- Cholesterol 73 mg
- Sodium 346 mg
- Total Carbohydrate 25 g
- Dietary Fiber 4 g
- Protein 26 g
- Total Sugars 9 g
- Potassium 545 mg

Garlic Pork Loin

Preparation Time: 15 minutes
Cooking Time: 1 hour
Servings: 6

Ingredients:

- 1 ½ lb. pork loin roast
- 4 cloves garlic, sliced into slivers
- Salt and pepper to taste

Method:

1. Preheat your oven to 425 degrees F.
2. Make several slits all over the pork roast.
3. Insert garlic slivers.
4. Sprinkle with salt and pepper.
5. Roast in the oven for 1 hour.

Nutritional Value:

- Calories 235
- Total Fat 13.3 g
- Saturated Fat 2.6 g
- Cholesterol 71 mg
- Sodium 450 mg
- Total Carbohydrate 1.7 g
- Dietary Fiber 0.3 g
- Protein 25.7 g
- Total Sugars 3 g
- Potassium 383 mg

Chapter 5: Chicken Recipes

Chicken with Red Pepper Sauce

Preparation Time: 20 minutes
Cooking Time: 20 minutes
Servings: 4

Ingredients:

- 1 tomato
- 2 red bell peppers
- 1 lb. chicken cutlets
- Salt and pepper to taste
- 2 tablespoons olive oil
- 1 clove garlic
- ½ cup pecans, toasted and chopped
- ¼ teaspoon red pepper flakes
- 1 tablespoon red-wine vinegar
- Chopped chives

Method:

1. Preheat your grill.
2. Grill the tomato and red bell peppers for 5 minutes per side.
3. Put the grilled veggies on a plate and let cool.
4. Season both sides of chicken with salt and pepper.
5. Grill for 4 to 5 minutes per side.
6. Let cool on a plate.
7. Peel the veggies and transfer to a blender.
8. Add the rest of the ingredients.
9. Pulse until smooth.
10. Spread the red pepper sauce on top of the chicken and serve.

Nutritional Value:

- Calories 308
- Total Fat 19.7 g
- Saturated Fat 2.6 g
- Cholesterol 63 mg

- Sodium 496 mg
- Total Carbohydrate 6 g
- Dietary Fiber 3.2 g
- Protein 25 g
- Total Sugars 4 g
- Potassium 471 mg

Chicken Pesto

Preparation Time: 15 minutes
Cooking Time: 25 minutes
Servings: 4

Ingredients:

- 1 lb. chicken cutlet
- Salt and pepper to taste
- 1 tablespoon olive oil
- ½ cup onion, chopped
- ½ cup heavy cream
- ½ cup dry white wine
- 1 tomato, chopped
- ¼ cup pesto
- 2 tablespoons basil, chopped

Method:

1. Season chicken with salt and pepper.
2. Pour oil into a pan over medium heat.
3. Cook chicken for 3 to 4 minutes per side.
4. Place the chicken on a plate.
5. Add the onion to the pan.
6. Cook for 1 minute.
7. Stir in the rest of the ingredients.
8. Bring to a boil.
9. Simmer for 15 minutes.
10. Put the chicken back to the pan.
11. Cook for 2 more minutes and then serve.

Nutritional Value:

- Calories 371
- Total Fat 23.7 g
- Saturated Fat 9.2 g
- Cholesterol 117 mg
- Sodium 361 mg
- Total Carbohydrate 5.7 g

- Dietary Fiber 1 g
- Protein 27.7 g
- Total Sugars 3 g
- Potassium 567 mg

Roasted Chicken with Carrots

Preparation Time: 15 minutes
Cooking Time: 30 minutes
Servings: 8

Ingredients:

- 1 whole chicken, sliced into parts
- 2 tablespoons olive oil, divided
- 4 cloves garlic, minced and divided
- Salt and pepper to taste
- 1 lb. baby carrots
- ½ cup basil, chopped
- ½ cup parsley, chopped
- 2 tablespoons lemon juice
- 1 tablespoon capers, rinsed and drained
- 1 teaspoon anchovy paste
- 1 tablespoon water

Method:

1. Preheat your oven to 500 degrees F.
2. In a bowl, combine half of oil, half of garlic, salt and pepper.
3. Rub mixture all over the chicken.
4. Place the chicken in a baking pan surrounded with carrots.
5. Roast the chicken and carrots at 450 degrees F for 30 minutes.
6. Add the rest of the ingredients along with half of oil and half of garlic in a food processor.
7. Pulse until pureed.
8. Serve roasted chicken and carrots with herb sauce.

Nutritional Value:

- Calories 263
- Total Fat 17.7 g
- Saturated Fat 6 g
- Cholesterol 118 mg
- Sodium 361 mg
- Total Carbohydrate 11.1 g

- Dietary Fiber 3.2 g
- Protein 29.7 g
- Total Sugars 5 g
- Potassium 651 mg

Spicy Grilled Chicken

Preparation Time: 5 minutes
Cooking Time: 12 minutes
Servings: 4

Ingredients:

- 3 tablespoons olive oil
- 1 ½ teaspoons dried marjoram
- 2 teaspoons ground cumin
- ¼ teaspoon cayenne pepper
- ¼ teaspoon ground allspice
- Salt to taste
- 1 lb. chicken breast, trimmed

Method:

1. Preheat your grill.
2. Combine all the ingredients except chicken breast.
3. Coat the chicken with the mixture evenly.
4. Grill the chicken for 5 to 6 minutes per side. Let cool and slice.

Nutritional Value:

- Calories 341
- Total Fat 21.1 g
- Saturated Fat 3.2 g
- Cholesterol 83 mg
- Sodium 522 mg
- Total Carbohydrate 8.5 g
- Dietary Fiber 3.3 g
- Protein 28.3 g
- Total Sugars 3 g
- Potassium 711 mg

Chicken Cutlets

Preparation Time: 20 minutes
Cooking Time: 35 minutes
Servings: 4

Ingredients:

- 1 lb. chicken cutlets
- Salt and pepper to taste
- 1 tablespoon olive oil
- ½ cup onion, chopped
- 1 tomato, chopped
- ½ cup heavy cream
- ½ cup dry white wine

Method:

1. Season chicken with salt and pepper.
2. Pour oil into a pan over medium heat.
3. Cook chicken for 3 to 4 minutes per side.
4. Let cool on a plate.
5. Cook onion in the pan for 1 minute.
6. Add the remaining ingredients to the pan.
7. Put the chicken back to the pan.
8. Bring to a boil.
9. Simmer for 15 minutes.

Nutritional Value:

- Calories 331
- Total Fat 17.3 g
- Saturated Fat 8 g
- Cholesterol 117 mg
- Sodium 208 mg
- Total Carbohydrate 8.1 g
- Dietary Fiber 2.4 g
- Protein 28.6 g
- Total Sugars 4 g
- Potassium 906 mg

Baked Chicken

Preparation Time: 15 minutes
Cooking Time: 15 minutes
Servings: 4

Ingredients:

- 1 lb. chicken cutlets
- Pepper to taste
- 2 tablespoons olive oil
- ⅓ cup salami, chopped
- ¼ cup pepperoncini, chopped
- 2 tablespoons red-wine vinegar
- 1 tablespoon fresh oregano, chopped
- 2 oz. fresh mozzarella cheese, grated

Method:

1. Preheat your broiler.
2. Season chicken with pepper.
3. In a bowl, combine the remaining ingredients except the mozzarella.
4. Cook the chicken in a pan over medium heat for 3 to 4 minutes per side.
5. Transfer to a baking pan poured with the mixture.
6. Bake for 3 minutes.
7. Sprinkle cheese on top.
8. Bake for another 2 minutes.

Nutritional Value:

- Calories 303
- Total Fat 19.6 g
- Saturated Fat 5 g
- Cholesterol 82 mg
- Sodium 476 mg
- Total Carbohydrate 2.8 g
- Dietary Fiber 0.7 g
- Protein 27.6 g
- Total Sugars 3 g
- Potassium 263 mg

Chicken Kurma

Preparation Time: 20 minutes
Cooking Time: 25 minutes
Servings: 6

Ingredients:

- 1 tablespoon olive oil
- 1 onion, diced
- 3 cloves garlic, sliced thinly
- 1 ginger, minced
- 2 tomatoes, diced
- 1 serrano pepper, minced
- Salt and pepper to taste
- 1 teaspoon ground turmeric
- 1 tablespoon tomato paste
- 1 ½ lb. chicken, sliced
- 1 red bell pepper, chopped

Method:

1. Pour oil into a pan over medium heat.
2. Cook onion for 3 minutes.
3. Add garlic, ginger, tomatoes, Serrano pepper, salt, pepper, turmeric and tomato paste.
4. Bring to a boil.
5. Reduce heat and simmer for 10 minutes.
6. Add chicken and cook for 5 minutes.
7. Stir in red bell pepper.
8. Cook for 5 minutes.

Nutritional Value:

- Calories 175
- Total Fat 15.2 g
- Saturated Fat 3 g
- Cholesterol 115 mg
- Sodium 400 mg
- Total Carbohydrate 7 g

- Dietary Fiber 1.8 g
- Protein 24 g
- Total Sugars 3 g
- Potassium 436 mg

Baked Lemon & Pepper Chicken

Preparation Time: 20 minutes
Cooking Time: 25 minutes
Servings: 4

Ingredients:

- 4 chicken breast fillets
- Salt to taste
- 1 tablespoon olive oil
- 1 lemon, sliced thinly
- 1 tablespoon maple syrup
- 2 tablespoons lemon juice
- 2 tablespoons butter
- Pepper to taste

Method:

1. Preheat your oven to 425 degrees F.
2. Season chicken with salt.
3. Pour oil into a pan over medium heat.
4. Cook chicken for 5 minutes per side.
5. Transfer chicken to a baking pan.
6. Surround the chicken with the lemon slices.
7. Bake in the oven for 10 minutes.
8. Pour in maple syrup and lemon juice to the pan.
9. Put the butter on top of the chicken.
10. Sprinkle with pepper.
11. Bake for another 5 minutes.

Nutritional Value:

- Calories 286
- Total Fat 13 g
- Saturated Fat 5 g
- Cholesterol 109 mg
- Sodium 448 mg
- Total Carbohydrate 7 g
- Dietary Fiber 1.4 g
- Protein 34.8 g
- Total Sugars 3 g
- Potassium 350 mg

Garlic Parmesan Chicken Wings

Preparation Time: 20 minutes
Cooking Time: 20 minutes
Servings: 8

Ingredients:

- Cooking spray
- ½ cup all-purpose flour
- Pepper to taste
- 2 tablespoons garlic powder
- 3 eggs, beaten
- 1 ¼ cups Parmesan cheese, grated
- 2 cups breadcrumbs
- 2 lb. chicken wings

Method:

1. Preheat your oven to 450 degrees F.
2. Spray baking pan with oil.
3. In a bowl, mix the flour, pepper and garlic powder.
4. Add eggs to another bowl.
5. Mix the Parmesan cheese and breadcrumbs in another bowl.
6. Dip the chicken wings in the first, second and third bowls.
7. Spray chicken wings with oil.
8. Bake in the oven for 20 minutes.

Nutritional Value:

- Calories 221
- Total Fat 11.6 g
- Saturated Fat 3.9 g
- Cholesterol 122 mg
- Sodium 242 mg
- Total Carbohydrate 8 g
- Dietary Fiber 0.4 g
- Protein 16 g
- Total Sugars 3 g
- Potassium 163 mg

Chicken Paprika

Preparation Time: 20 minutes
Cooking Time: 15 minutes
Servings: 4

Ingredients:

- 1 lb. chicken cutlets
- Salt and pepper to taste
- 2 tablespoons olive oil, divided
- 1 onion, sliced
- 8 oz. white mushrooms, sliced
- 4 teaspoons sweet paprika
- ¼ teaspoon red pepper flakes
- ½ cup chicken broth
- ½ cup sour cream
- Chopped parsley

Method:

1. Season chicken with salt and pepper.
2. Pour half of oil into a pan over medium heat.
3. Cook chicken for 3 minutes per side.
4. Let cool on a plate.
5. Add remaining oil to a pan.
6. Cook onion for 5 minutes.
7. Stir in the mushrooms and the rest of the ingredients to the pan.
8. Bring to a simmer for 5 minutes.
9. Return chicken to the pan.
10. Cook for 2 minutes and serve.

Nutritional Value:

- Calories 282
- Total Fat 15 g
- Saturated Fat 4 g
- Cholesterol 97 mg
- Sodium 365 mg
- Total Carbohydrate 5 g

- Dietary Fiber 1.6 g
- Protein 28 g
- Total Sugars 4 g
- Potassium 780 mg

Chapter 6: Seafood Recipes

Crunchy Walleye

Preparation Time: 15 minutes
Cooking Time: 15 minutes
Servings: 4

Ingredients:

Tartar Sauce

- ½ cup mayonnaise
- 1 clove garlic, minced
- ⅓ cup fresh dill, chopped
- 1 tablespoon lemon juice
- 1 teaspoon lemon zest
- Pepper to taste

Fish

- 1 teaspoon Old Bay seasoning
- ¼ cup all-purpose flour
- 1 egg, beaten
- ¼ cup milk
- 1 cup whole-wheat breadcrumbs
- 4 walleye fillets
- Salt to taste
- 4 tablespoons olive oil

Method:

1. Mix tartar sauce ingredients in a bowl and set aside.
2. In a plate, mix Old Bay seasoning and flour.
3. In another plate, blend egg and milk.
4. Put the breadcrumbs in a third plate.
5. Season fish fillets with salt.
6. Dip the fish fillets in the first, second and third plates.
7. Pour oil into a pan over medium heat.
8. Fry the fish until crispy.

9. Serve fish with tartar sauce.

Nutritional Value:

- Calories 454
- Total Fat 37 g
- Saturated Fat 8 g
- Cholesterol 87 mg
- Sodium 471 mg
- Total Carbohydrate 7 g
- Dietary Fiber 1 g
- Protein 17 g
- Total Sugars 2 g
- Potassium 349 mg

Salmon Cakes

Preparation Time: 15 minutes
Cooking Time: 10 minutes
Servings: 4

Ingredients:

- 1 lb. salmon flakes
- 1 red bell pepper, chopped
- 1 tablespoon lemon juice
- 2 teaspoons Dijon mustard
- 1 tablespoon shallot, chopped
- ¼ cup buttermilk
- ½ cup panko breadcrumbs
- Salt and pepper to taste
- 3 tablespoons chopped fresh dill
- Olive oil

Method:

1. Add all ingredients except olive e oil to a bowl.
2. Mix well.
3. Form patties from the mixture.
4. Fry the patties in olive oil for 3 to 5 minutes per side or until golden.

Nutritional Value:

- Calories 424
- Total Fat 26.7 g
- Saturated Fat 9.4 g
- Cholesterol 97 mg
- Sodium 494 mg
- Total Carbohydrate 13.9 g
- Dietary Fiber 1.6 g
- Protein 29.8 g
- Total Sugars 4 g
- Potassium 923 mg

Crispy Cod with Herbed Cream Sauce

Preparation Time: 15 minutes
Cooking Time: 10 minutes
Servings: 4

Ingredients:

- 2 tablespoons buttermilk
- 2 tablespoons mayonnaise
- 1 tablespoon dill, chopped
- 1 tablespoon chives, chopped
- 1 tablespoon basil, chopped
- Salt and pepper to taste
- 1 ¼ lb. cod fillet, sliced into strips
- 2 tablespoon whole-wheat flour
- 2 tablespoons olive oil

Method:

1. Combine milk, mayo, herbs, salt and pepper in a bowl. Set aside.
2. Season fish with salt and pepper.
3. Dredge with flour.
4. Pour the oil into a pan over medium heat.
5. Cook for 3 to 4 minutes per side or until crispy.
6. Pour the sauce over the fish and serve.

Nutritional Value:

- Calories 270
- Total Fat 12.9 g
- Saturated Fat 1.7 g
- Cholesterol 57 mg
- Sodium 462 mg
- Total Carbohydrate 7 g
- Dietary Fiber 3 g
- Protein 25 g
- Total Sugars 4 g
- Potassium 264 mg

Crispy Baked Shrimp

Preparation Time: 15 minutes
Cooking Time: 10 minutes
Servings: 4

Ingredients:

- ¼ cup whole-wheat breadcrumbs
- 3 tablespoons olive oil, divided
- 1 ½ lb. jumbo shrimp, peeled and deveined
- Salt and pepper to taste
- 2 tablespoons lemon juice
- 1 tablespoon garlic, chopped
- 2 tablespoons butter
- ¼ cup Parmesan cheese, grated
- 2 tablespoons chives, chopped

Method:

1. Preheat your oven to 425 degrees F.
2. Add breadcrumbs to a pan over medium heat.
3. Cook until toasted.
4. Transfer to a plate.
5. Coat baking pan with 1 tablespoon oil.
6. Arrange shrimp in a single layer in a baking pan.
7. Season with salt and pepper.
8. Mix lemon juice, garlic and butter in a bowl.
9. Pour mixture on top of the shrimp.
10. Add Parmesan cheese and chives to the breadcrumbs.
11. Sprinkle breadcrumbs on top of the shrimp.
12. Bake for 10 minutes.

Nutritional Value:

- Calories 340
- Total Fat 18.7 g
- Saturated Fat 6 g
- Cholesterol 293 mg
- Sodium 374 mg

- Total Carbohydrate 6 g
- Dietary Fiber 0.8 g
- Protein 36.9 g
- Total Sugars 2 g
- Potassium 483 mg

Baked Tuna Steak

Preparation Time: 20 minutes
Cooking Time: 15 minutes
Servings: 4

Ingredients:

- 4 tuna steaks
- Salt and pepper to taste
- ¼ cup mayonnaise
- 1 teaspoon honey
- 2 teaspoons Dijon mustard
- 1 tablespoon fresh parsley, chopped
- ½ teaspoon ground turmeric

Method:

1. Preheat your oven to 450 degrees F.
2. Season tuna steaks with salt and pepper.
3. In a bowl, mix the remaining ingredients.
4. Place the tuna steaks on top of a foil sheet.
5. Spread the mixture on top of the fish.
6. Fold the foil and seal.
7. Bake in the oven for 15 minutes.

Nutritional Value:

- Calories 312
- Total Fat 11.3 g
- Saturated Fat 1.9 g
- Cholesterol 61 mg
- Sodium 512 mg
- Total Carbohydrate 14 g
- Dietary Fiber 1.7 g
- Protein 36.4 g
- Total Sugars 2 g
- Potassium 901 mg

Lemon & Rosemary Salmon

Preparation Time: 10 minutes
Cooking Time: 15 minutes
Servings: 4

Ingredients:

- 4 salmon fillets
- Salt and pepper to taste
- 4 tablespoons butter
- 1 lemon, sliced
- 8 rosemary sprigs

Method:

1. Season salmon with salt and pepper.
2. Place salmon on a foil sheet.
3. Top with butter, lemon slices and rosemary sprigs.
4. Fold the foil and seal.
5. Bake in the oven at 450 degrees F for 15 minutes.

Nutritional Value:

- Calories 365
- Total Fat 22 g
- Saturated Fat 6 g
- Cholesterol 86 mg
- Sodium 445 mg
- Total Carbohydrate 5 g
- Dietary Fiber 1.9 g
- Protein 29.8 g
- Total Sugars 3 g
- Potassium 782 mg

Mediterranean Fish

Preparation Time: 20 minutes
Cooking Time: 20 minutes
Servings: 4

Ingredients:

- 3 tablespoons olive oil, divided
- 1 onion, sliced
- 2 cloves garlic, sliced
- 3 cups mushrooms, sliced
- 1 tomato, diced
- 4 cups kale, chopped
- 2 teaspoons Mediterranean herb mix, divided
- 1 tablespoon lemon juice
- Salt and pepper to taste
- 4 fish fillets

Method:

1. Pour 1 tablespoon oil into a pan over medium heat.
2. Cook onion, garlic and mushrooms for 5 minutes.
3. Stir in tomato and kale.
4. Season with half of herb mix.
5. Pour lemon juice and season with salt and pepper.
6. Simmer for 5 minutes.
7. Transfer to a plate.
8. Season fish fillet with salt and pepper.
9. Add remaining oil to the pan.
10. Cook fish for 3 to 4 minutes per side.
11. Serve fish poured with the veggies and sauce.

Nutritional Value:

- Calories 214
- Total Fat 11 g
- Saturated Fat 2 g
- Cholesterol 45 mg
- Sodium 598 mg

- Total Carbohydrate 11 g
- Dietary Fiber 3 g
- Protein 18 g
- Total Sugars 4 g
- Potassium 736 mg

Roasted Salmon Caprese

Preparation Time: 20 minutes
Cooking Time: 10 minutes
Servings: 4

Ingredients:

- 1 teaspoon olive oil
- 1 clove garlic, minced
- Salt and pepper to taste
- 2 cups cherry tomatoes, sliced
- 4 salmon fillets
- 4 tablespoons mozzarella, shredded
- ¼ cup basil, chopped
- 2 teaspoons balsamic glaze

Method:

1. Preheat your oven to 425 degrees F.
2. In a bowl, mix the olive oil, salt and pepper.
3. Place the fish in a baking pan.
4. Top with the mozzarella and basil.
5. Bake for 10 minutes.
6. Drizzle fish with balsamic glaze and serve with tomatoes.

Nutritional Value:

- Calories 291
- Total Fat 18.2 g
- Saturated Fat 4.4 g
- Cholesterol 67 mg
- Sodium 406 mg
- Total Carbohydrate 5.2 g
- Dietary Fiber 1.1 g
- Protein 25.8 g
- Total Sugars 3 g
- Potassium 617 mg

Herbed Mediterranean Fish Fillet

Preparation Time: 20 minutes
Cooking Time: 1 hour
Servings: 6

Ingredients:

- 3 lb. sea bass fillet
- Salt to taste
- 2 tablespoons tarragon, chopped
- ¼ cup dry white wine
- 3 tablespoons olive oil, divided
- 1 tablespoon butter
- 2 cloves garlic, minced
- 2 cups whole-wheat breadcrumbs
- 3 tablespoons parsley, chopped
- 3 tablespoons oregano, chopped
- 3 tablespoons fresh basil, chopped

Method:

1. Preheat your oven to 350 degrees F.
2. Season fish with salt and tarragon.
3. Pour half of oil into a roasting pan.
4. Stir in wine.
5. Add the fish in the roasting pan.
6. Bake in the oven for 50 minutes.
7. Add remaining oil to a pan over medium heat.
8. Cook herbs, breadcrumbs and salt.
9. Spread breadcrumb mixture on top of fish and bake for 5 minutes.

Nutritional Value:

- Calories 288
- Total Fat 12.7 g
- Saturated Fat 2.9 g
- Cholesterol 65 mg
- Sodium 499 mg
- Total Carbohydrate 10.4 g

- Dietary Fiber 1.8 g
- Protein 29.5 g
- Total Sugars 1 g
- Potassium 401 mg

Honey Shrimp

Preparation Time: 10 minutes
Cooking Time: 5 minutes
Servings: 4

Ingredients:

- 2 tablespoons water
- 2 tablespoons light brown sugar
- 1 lb. shrimp, peeled and deveined
- 1 tablespoon honey
- 2 tablespoons extra-virgin olive oil, divided
- 3 tablespoons mayonnaise
- 1 tablespoon lemon juice
- Salt and pepper to taste
- ½ cup scallions, sliced

Method:

1. Pour water into a pan over medium heat.
2. Stir in brown sugar.
3. Cook for 2 minutes.
4. Pour into a bowl.
5. Add shrimp to the pan.
6. Cook for 3 minutes, stirring.
7. In a bowl, mix the remaining ingredients.
8. Pour brown sugar mixture over the fish and serve with the sauce.

Nutritional Value:

- Calories 358
- Total Fat 23.6 g
- Saturated Fat 3 g
- Cholesterol 186 mg
- Sodium 193 mg
- Total Carbohydrate 8.7 g
- Dietary Fiber 1.4 g
- Protein 25.4 g
- Total Sugars 11 g
- Potassium 411 mg

Chapter 7: Vegetarian Recipes

Tofu & Mushroom Stir Fry

Preparation Time: 15 minutes
Cooking Time: 10 minutes
Servings: 5

Ingredients:

- 4 tablespoons olive oil, divided
- 1 red bell pepper, diced
- 1 lb. mushrooms, sliced
- 1 clove garlic, grated
- 1 tablespoon ginger, grated
- 1 cup scallions, chopped
- 8 oz. tofu, diced
- 3 tablespoons oyster sauce

Method:

1. Add half of oil to a pan over medium heat.
2. Cook bell pepper and mushrooms for 4 minutes.
3. Stir in garlic, ginger and scallions for 1 minute.
4. Transfer to a bowl.
5. Pour the remaining oil to the pan.
6. Cook the tofu for 4 minutes or until golden.
7. Drain the oil.
8. Add the veggies and oyster sauce to the pan.
9. Cook for 1 minute.

Nutritional Value:

- Calories 171
- Total Fat 13.1 g
- Saturated Fat 2.3 g
- Cholesterol 102 mg
- Sodium 309 mg
- Total Carbohydrate 8.6 g
- Dietary Fiber 2.3 g

- Protein 7.7 g
- Total Sugars 3 g
- Potassium 469 mg

Lettuce Wrap

Preparation Time: 20 minutes
Cooking Time: 30 minutes
Servings: 4

Ingredients:

- 1 teaspoon sesame oil
- 2 tablespoons soy sauce
- 2 tablespoons hoisin sauce
- 3 tablespoons rice vinegar
- ¼ teaspoon red pepper flakes
- 1 tablespoon olive oil
- 14 oz. tofu, sliced into cubes
- 1 tablespoon ginger, grated
- 3 cloves garlic, minced
- 8 oz. mushrooms, chopped
- 4 scallions, chopped
- 8 lettuce leaves

Method:

1. Mix sesame oil, soy sauce, hoisin sauce, vinegar and red pepper flakes in a bowl. Set aside.
2. Add olive oil to a pan over medium heat.
3. Cook tofu until golden.
4. Stir in the ginger, garlic, mushrooms and scallions.
5. Pour in sauce.
6. Simmer for 15 minutes.
7. Put mixture on top of the lettuce leaves.
8. Roll up the lettuce leaves and serve.

Nutritional Value:

- Calories 178
- Total Fat 10.9 g
- Saturated Fat 1.4 g
- Cholesterol 125 mg
- Sodium 408 mg

- Total Carbohydrate 10.6 g
- Dietary Fiber 1.9 g
- Protein 12.9 g
- Total Sugars 5 g
- Potassium 517 mg

Eggplant Pizza

Preparation Time: 20 minutes
Cooking Time: 20 minutes
Servings: 4

Ingredients:

- 1 lb. eggplant, sliced thickly
- Salt and pepper to taste
- 2 tablespoons olive oil
- ¼ cup marinara sauce
- 1 cup mushrooms, sliced and cooked
- 2 oz. turkey sausage, removed from casing and cooked
- 1 cup mozzarella cheese, shredded
- 2 tablespoons fresh basil, chopped

Method:

1. Preheat your oven to 375 degrees F.
2. Season eggplant with salt.
3. Let sit for 10 minutes.
4. Dry with paper towel.
5. Brush with oil and season with pepper.
6. Arrange in a single layer in a baking pan.
7. Bake for 20 minutes.
8. Spread marinara sauce on top of eggplant.
9. Top with the mushrooms, sausage, cheese and basil.

Nutritional Value:

- Calories 214
- Total Fat 19.4 g
- Saturated Fat 8.6 g
- Cholesterol 32 mg
- Sodium 453 mg
- Total Carbohydrate 7 g
- Dietary Fiber 3.7 g
- Protein 12 g
- Total Sugars 6 g
- Potassium 491 mg

Roasted Tofu in Lime Sauce with Green Beans

Preparation Time: 1 hour and 15 minutes
Cooking Time: 20 minutes
Servings: 4

Ingredients:

- 6 tablespoons sesame oil
- ¼ cup soy sauce
- ¼ cup lime juice
- 28 oz. tofu, sliced into cubes
- Steamed green beans

Method:

1. Mix sesame oil, soy sauce and lime juice in a bowl.
2. Add the tofu cubes.
3. Marinate for 1 hour.
4. Preheat your oven to 450 degrees F.
5. Spread the tofu in a baking pan.
6. Roast for 20 minutes.

Nutritional Value:

- Calories 163
- Total Fat 14.6 g
- Saturated Fat 5 g
- Cholesterol 20 mg
- Sodium 111 mg
- Total Carbohydrate 2 g
- Dietary Fiber 1.9 g
- Protein 19 g
- Total Sugars 1 g
- Potassium 30 mg

Mushroom Stuffed with Ricotta

Preparation Time: 10 minutes
Cooking Time: 10 minutes
Servings: 4

Ingredients:

- 4 large mushrooms, stemmed
- 1 tablespoon olive oil
- Salt and pepper to taste
- ¼ cup basil, chopped
- 1 cup ricotta cheese
- ¼ cup Parmesan cheese, grated

Method:

1. Preheat your grill.
2. Coat the mushrooms with oil.
3. Season with salt and pepper.
4. Grill for 5 minutes.
5. Stuff each mushroom with a mixture of basil, ricotta cheese and Parmesan cheese.
6. Grill for another 5 minutes.

Nutritional Value:

- Calories 259
- Total Fat 17.3 g
- Saturated Fat 5.4 g
- Cholesterol 24 mg
- Sodium 509 mg
- Total Carbohydrate 14.9 g
- Dietary Fiber 2.6 g
- Protein 12.2 g
- Total Sugars 7 g
- Potassium 572 mg

Cucumber & Honeydew Salad

Preparation Time: 15 minutes
Cooking Time: 0 minutes
Servings: 6

Ingredients:

- 2 tablespoons olive oil
- 3 tablespoons lemon juice
- ¼ cup fresh basil, chopped
- 1 ½ teaspoons honey
- Salt and pepper to taste
- 4 cups baby arugula
- 4 cups honeydew melon, sliced into cubes
- 2 cucumbers, chopped
- ¼ cup pepitas, toasted

Method:

1. Combine olive oil, lemon juice, honey, basil, salt and pepper in a bowl.
2. In a salad bowl, arrange the baby arugula and top with the cucumber and melon.
3. Drizzle with the dressing.
4. Sprinkle pepitas on top.

Nutritional Value:

- Calories 171
- Total Fat 14 g
- Saturated Fat 5 g
- Cholesterol 13 mg
- Sodium 188 mg
- Total Carbohydrate 4.6 g
- Dietary Fiber 1.7 g
- Protein 5.9 g
- Total Sugars 12 g
- Potassium 370 mg

Caprese Salad with Avocado

Preparation Time: 15 minutes
Cooking Time: 0 minutes
Servings: 6

Ingredients:

- 1 tablespoon balsamic vinegar
- 2 tablespoons olive oil
- Salt and pepper to taste
- 2 cups baby arugula
- 1 cup avocado, sliced into cubes
- 4 cups tomatoes, sliced

Method:

1. Mix vinegar, oil, salt and pepper in a bowl.
2. Toss the baby arugula in the mixture.
3. Arrange on a platter.
4. Top with the avocado cubes and tomatoes.

Nutritional Value:

- Calories 116
- Total Fat 18 g
- Saturated Fat 7 g
- Cholesterol 14 mg
- Sodium 260 mg
- Total Carbohydrate 5.6 g
- Dietary Fiber 1.6 g
- Protein 4.8 g
- Total Sugars 4 g
- Potassium 328 mg

Roasted Brussels Sprouts with Goat Cheese

Preparation Time: 15 minutes
Cooking Time: 20 minutes
Servings: 4

Ingredients:

- 1 lb. Brussels sprouts, sliced in half
- 1 shallot, chopped
- 1 tablespoons olive oil
- Salt and pepper to taste
- 2 teaspoons balsamic vinegar
- ¼ cup goat cheese, crumbled

Method:

1. Preheat your oven to 400 degrees F.
2. Coat the Brussels sprouts with oil, salt and pepper.
3. Spread Brussels sprouts in the baking pan.
4. Roast for 20 minutes.
5. Drizzle with vinegar and sprinkle goat cheese on top.

Nutritional Value:

- Calories 117
- Total Fat 7 g
- Saturated Fat 3 g
- Cholesterol 4 mg
- Sodium 216 mg
- Total Carbohydrate 13 g
- Dietary Fiber 4.8 g
- Protein 5.8 g
- Total Sugars 5 g
- Potassium 491 mg

Thai Chopped Salad

Preparation Time: 15 minutes
Cooking Time: 0 minutes
Servings: 4

Ingredients:

- 10 oz. kale and cabbage mix
- 14 oz. tofu, sliced into cubes and fried crispy
- ½ cup vinaigrette

Method:

1. Arrange kale and cabbage in a serving platter.
2. Top with the tofu cubes.
3. Drizzle with the vinaigrette.

Nutritional Value:

- Calories 332
- Total Fat 15 g
- Saturated Fat 1.5 g
- Cholesterol 0 mg
- Sodium 236 mg
- Total Carbohydrate 26.3 g
- Dietary Fiber 7.6 g
- Protein 1.3 g
- Total Sugars 13 g
- Potassium 41 mg

Avocados with Yogurt

Preparation Time: 15 minutes
Cooking Time: 0 minutes
Servings: 4

Ingredients:

- ½ cup Greek yogurt
- 2 teaspoons mayonnaise
- 1 tablespoon lime juice
- 1 teaspoon Dijon mustard
- 2 tablespoons parsley, chopped
- Salt and pepper to taste
- 2 avocado, sliced in half and pitted
- Chopped chives

Method:

1. Mix yogurt, mayonnaise, lime juice, mustard, parsley, salt and pepper.
2. Stuff avocado with the mixture.
3. Garnish with chives.

Nutritional Value:

- Calories 293
- Total Fat 19.3 g
- Saturated Fat 3 g
- Cholesterol 61 mg
- Sodium 400 mg
- Total Carbohydrate 10.5 g
- Dietary Fiber 7 g
- Protein 22.5 g
- Total Sugars 2 g
- Potassium 807 mg

Chapter 8: Snacks and Desserts Recipes

Smoky Pumpkin Seeds

Preparation Time: 10 minutes
Cooking Time: 40 minutes
Servings: 8

Ingredients:

- 2 tablespoons olive oil
- 1 teaspoon garlic powder
- 1 teaspoon dried oregano
- 2 teaspoons smoked paprika
- Salt to taste
- 2 cups pumpkin seeds

Method:

1. Preheat your oven to 300 degrees F.
2. In a bowl, mix the olive oil, garlic powder, dried oregano, smoked paprika and salt.
3. Coat the pumpkin seeds in this mixture.
4. Spread seeds in a baking pan.
5. Bake for 40 minutes.

Nutritional Value:

- Calories 215
- Total Fat 17.6 g
- Saturated Fat 4 g
- Cholesterol 102 mg
- Sodium 151 mg
- Total Carbohydrate 4.7 g
- Dietary Fiber 3.3 g
- Protein 9.2 g
- Total Sugars 1 g
- Potassium 19 mg

Kale Chips

Preparation Time: 10 minutes
Cooking Time: 10 minutes
Servings: 2

Ingredients:

- Cooking spray
- 6 cups kale leaves, chopped
- 1 ½ teaspoons low-sodium soy sauce
- 1 tablespoon olive oil
- Salt to taste
- ¼ teaspoon ground cumin
- ½ teaspoon sesame seeds

Method:

1. Spray your baking pan with oil.
2. Mix the soy sauce, oil and salt in a bowl.
3. Coat the kale with this mixture.
4. Massage the kale.
5. Arrange the kale in a baking pan.
6. Bake at 375 degrees F for 10 minutes.
7. Sprinkle with cumin and sesame seeds.

Nutritional Value:

- Calories 140
- Total Fat 9.4 g
- Saturated Fat 1.2 g
- Cholesterol 20 mg
- Sodium 329 mg
- Total Carbohydrate 12.8 g
- Dietary Fiber 4.4 g
- Protein 5 g
- Total Sugars 3 g
- Potassium 497 mg

Fruit Balls

Preparation Time: 45 minutes
Cooking Time: 0 minutes
Servings: 20

Ingredients:

- 1 cup dried apricots
- 1 cup dried figs
- 1 cup almonds, chopped
- ¼ cup coconut flakes, shredded

Method:

1. Add apricots, figs and almonds to a blender.
2. Pulse until chopped finely.
3. Form balls from the mixture.
4. Dredge with coconut flakes.
5. Refrigerate for 30 minutes.

Nutritional Value:

- Calories 70
- Total Fat 3.3 g
- Saturated Fat 0.9 g
- Cholesterol 100 mg
- Sodium 2 mg
- Total Carbohydrate 10 g
- Dietary Fiber 2 g
- Protein 7 g
- Total Sugars 7 g
- Potassium 167 mg

Peach Muffins

Preparation Time: 15 minutes
Cooking Time: 10 minutes
Servings: 25

Ingredients:

- 2 cups all-purpose flour
- ¼ teaspoon salt
- 1 ½ teaspoons baking powder
- 1 cup sugar
- ⅔ cup milk
- 3 oz. cream cheese
- 3 tablespoons Greek yogurt
- 1 egg
- 3 tablespoons canola oil
- 2 cups peach slices
- ¼ teaspoon ground cinnamon
- 2 tablespoons butter

Method:

1. Preheat your oven to 375 degrees F.
2. In a bowl, combine flour, salt and baking powder.
3. Use a mixer to beat sugar, milk, cream cheese and yogurt.
4. Stir in egg and oil.
5. Slowly add flour mixture.
6. Fold in the peach slices.
7. Pour the batter into the muffin cups.
8. Bake for 10 minutes.
9. Let cool before serving.

Nutritional Value:

- Calories 156
- Total Fat 13 g
- Saturated Fat 7 g
- Cholesterol 10 mg
- Sodium 34 mg

- Total Carbohydrate 9 g
- Dietary Fiber 1 g
- Protein 1 g
- Total Sugars 5 g
- Potassium 221 mg

Crispy Chickpeas

Preparation Time: 15 minutes
Cooking Time: 15 minutes
Servings: 4

Ingredients:

- 15 oz. chickpeas, rinsed and drained
- 1 ½ tablespoons toasted sesame oil
- Salt to taste
- ¼ teaspoon smoked paprika
- ¼ teaspoon red pepper flakes
- Cooking spray

Method:

1. Coat the chickpeas with oil.
2. Season with salt, paprika and red pepper flakes.
3. Spray with oil.
4. Roast in the oven at 400 degrees F for 15 minutes.

Nutritional Value:

- Calories 132
- Total Fat 8 g
- Saturated Fat 2 g
- Cholesterol 10 mg
- Sodium 86 mg
- Total Carbohydrate 4 g
- Dietary Fiber 3.4 g
- Protein 4.7 g
- Total Sugars 86 g
- Potassium 152 mg

Avocado & Black Bean Dip

Preparation Time: 20 minutes
Cooking Time: 0 minutes
Servings: 12

Ingredients:

- 4 avocados
- 1 cup black beans, rinsed and drained
- 1 tablespoon lime juice
- 1 jalapeño pepper, chopped
- ½ teaspoon ground cumin
- 2 tablespoons fresh cilantro, chopped
- Salt and pepper to taste

Method:

1. Mashed the avocados and black beans in a bowl.
2. Stir in the rest of the ingredients.
3. Serve with keto crackers.

Nutritional Value:

- Calories 130
- Total Fat 10 g
- Saturated Fat 1.4 g
- Cholesterol 80 mg
- Sodium 152 mg
- Total Carbohydrate 10.2 g
- Dietary Fiber 5.6 g
- Protein 2.5 g
- Total Sugars 1 g
- Potassium 390 mg

Tomato Salsa

Preparation Time: 10 minutes
Cooking Time: 0 minutes
Servings: 12

Ingredients:

- 2 cups tomatoes, chopped
- 2 tablespoons white onion, chopped
- 1 clove garlic, minced
- 2 teaspoon marjoram, chopped
- Salt and pepper to taste

Method:

1. Add all the ingredients to a food processor.
2. Pulse until pureed.
3. Serve with keto chips.

Nutritional Value:

- Calories 55
- Total Fat 8 g
- Saturated Fat 3 g
- Cholesterol 0 mg
- Sodium 81 mg
- Total Carbohydrate 1 g
- Dietary Fiber 0.3 g
- Protein 3 g
- Total Sugars 1 g
- Potassium 58 mg

Pecan Muffins

Preparation Time: 20 minutes
Cooking Time: 20 minutes
Servings: 24

Ingredients:

- 1 ½ cups rolled oats
- Cooking spray
- ½ cup keto flour
- ½ cup keto sweetener
- Pinch salt
- 2 eggs
- 1 teaspoon vanilla extract
- 8 tablespoons butter, sliced into cubes
- ¼ cup maple syrup
- 1 cup pecans, chopped

Method:

1. Add rolled oats to a food processor.
2. Pulse until finely chopped.
3. Spray your muffin pan with oil.
4. Preheat your oven to 350 degrees F.
5. Add fine oats to a bowl.
6. Stir in the rest of the ingredients except butter, maple syrup and pecans.
7. Divide mixture among muffin cups.
8. Bake in the oven for 15 minutes.
9. Add the butter to a pan over medium heat.
10. Stir in maple syrup.
11. Pour mixture over the muffins and sprinkle with pecans.
12. Bake for another 5 minutes.

Nutritional Value:

- Calories 123
- Total Fat 7.6 g
- Saturated Fat 2.8 g
- Cholesterol 26 mg

- Sodium 105 mg
- Total Carbohydrate 3 g
- Dietary Fiber 1 g
- Protein 1.8 g
- Total Sugars 7 g
- Potassium 59 mg

Choco Chip Cookies

Preparation Time: 30 minutes
Cooking Time: 15 minutes
Servings: 24

Ingredients:

- 1 cup all-purpose flour
- ½ cup melted butter
- ½ cup almond flour
- ½ teaspoon salt
- 1 teaspoon baking soda
- 1 egg, beaten
- ⅓ cup brown sugar
- 1 teaspoon vanilla extract
- ¾ cup dark chocolate chips

Method:

1. Combine all the ingredients in a bowl.
2. Form cookies from the mixture.
3. Arrange in a baking pan.
4. Bake in the oven at 350 degrees F for 15 minutes.

Nutritional Value:

- Calories 118
- Total Fat 9.7 g
- Saturated Fat 3.3 g
- Cholesterol 18 mg
- Sodium 107 mg
- Total Carbohydrate 14 g
- Dietary Fiber 1 g
- Protein 1.6 g
- Total Sugars 6 g
- Potassium 53 mg

Blueberry Cobbler

Preparation Time: 15 minutes
Cooking Time: 30 minutes
Servings: 9

Ingredients:

- 1 tablespoon orange juice
- 2 tablespoons keto sweetener, divided
- 3 cups blueberries
- ¼ cup coconut flour
- ¾ cup almond flour
- ¼ teaspoon salt
- 4 tablespoons butter
- 1 teaspoon vanilla extract
- 1 egg, beaten

Method:

1. Preheat your oven to 375 degrees F.
2. Mix orange juice, half of sweetener and blueberries in a baking pan.
3. In a bowl, mix the remaining sweetener with the flours, salt and butter.
4. Stir in vanilla and egg.
5. Spread mixture on top of the blueberries.
6. Bake in the oven for 30 minutes.

Nutritional Value:

- Calories 161
- Total Fat 16 g
- Saturated Fat 8 g
- Cholesterol 34 mg
- Sodium 84 mg
- Total Carbohydrate 14 g
- Dietary Fiber 3.3 g
- Protein 3.6 g
- Total Sugars 8 g
- Potassium 51 mg

Chapter 9: 30-Day Meal plan

Day 1

Breakfast: Bacon, Mushroom and Spinach Quiches

Lunch: Garlic Pork Loin

Dinner: Lettuce Wrap

Day 2

Breakfast: Chaffle Sandwich with Bacon and Avocado

Lunch: Beef Bourguignon

Dinner: Caprese Salad with Avocado

Day 3

Breakfast: Cheesy Omelet with Bacon and Black Beans

Lunch: Baked Lemon and Pepper Chicken

Dinner: Pork Taco

Day 4

Breakfast: Toast with Raspberries & Mascarpone

Lunch: Crunchy Walleye

Dinner: Pork with Pears

Day 5

Breakfast: Cheesy Spinach and Broccoli Omelet

Lunch: Garlic Parmesan Chicken Wings

Dinner: Meatloaf with Sausage

Day 6

Breakfast: Omelet with Arugula and Tomatoes

Lunch: Salmon Cakes

Dinner: Cucumber and Honeydew Salad

Day 7

Breakfast: Omelet with Herbs and Goat Cheese

Lunch: Chicken Kurma

Dinner: Crispy Cod with Herbed Cream Sauce

Day 8

Breakfast: Cheesy Omelet with Bacon and Black Beans

Lunch: Rib Roast

Dinner: Roasted Tofu in Lime Sauce with Green Beans

Day 9

Breakfast: Omelet with Arugula and Tomatoes

Lunch: Chicken with Red Pepper Sauce

Dinner: Pork Tenderloin with Plum Chutney

Day 10

Breakfast: Keto Toast with Chicken and Cucumber

Lunch: Mushroom Stuffed with Ricotta

Dinner: Sweet and Spicy Flank Steak

Day 11

Breakfast: Greek Omelet with Feta

Lunch: Grilled Pork with Salsa

Dinner: Roasted Brussels Sprouts with Goat Cheese

Day 12

Breakfast: Chaffle Sandwich with Bacon and Avocado

Lunch: Grilled Steak with Tomato Salad

Dinner: Chicken Pesto

Day 13

Breakfast: Omelet with Sun-Dried Tomatoes and Sausage

Lunch: Mojo Pork

Dinner: Crispy Cod with Herbed Cream Sauce

Day 14

Breakfast: Cheesy Omelet with Bacon and Black Beans

Lunch: Beef Stir Fry

Dinner: Chicken with Red Pepper Sauce

Day 15

Breakfast: Bacon, Mushroom and Spinach Quiches

Lunch: Pork Braised in Wine

Dinner: Lettuce Wrap

Day 16

Breakfast: Omelet with Sun-Dried Tomatoes and Sausage

Lunch: Chicken Paprika

Dinner: Grilled Steak with Tomato Salad

Day 17

Breakfast: Cheesy Spinach & Broccoli Omelet

Lunch: Crunchy Walleye

Dinner: Chicken With Red Pepper Sauce

Day 18

Breakfast: Toast with Raspberries and Mascarpone

Lunch: Sweet and Sour Pork

Dinner: Eggplant Pizza

Day 19

Breakfast: Omelet with Herbs and Goat Cheese

Lunch: Roasted Chicken with Carrots

Dinner: Beef-Stuffed Mushrooms

Day 20

Breakfast: Chaffle Sandwich with Bacon and Avocado

Lunch: Crispy Baked Shrimp

Dinner: Prime Rib

Day 21

Breakfast: Toast with Raspberries and Mascarpone

Lunch: Crispy Cod with Herbed Cream Sauce

Dinner: Chicken Kurma

Day 22

Breakfast: Greek Omelet with Feta

Lunch: Honey Shrimp

Dinner: Herbed Mediterranean Fish Fillet

Day 23

Breakfast: Omelet with Sun-Dried Tomatoes and Sausage

Lunch: Beef Bourguignon

Dinner: Baked Tuna Steak

Day 24

Breakfast: Omelet with Arugula and Tomatoes

Lunch: Tofu and Mushroom Stir Fry

Dinner: Grilled Pork Tenderloin

Day 25

Breakfast: Bacon, Mushroom and Spinach Quiches

Lunch: Thai Chopped Salad

Dinner: Lemon and Rosemary Salmon

Day 26

Breakfast: Omelet with Herbs and Goat Cheese

Lunch: Seared Steak

Dinner: Spicy Grilled Chicken

Day 27

Breakfast: Cheesy Spinach and Broccoli Omelet

Lunch: Mediterranean Fish

Dinner: Tofu and Mushroom Stir Fry

Day 28

Breakfast: Greek Omelet with Feta

Lunch: Baked Chicken

Dinner: Beef-Stuffed Mushrooms

Day 29

Breakfast: Omelet with Arugula and Tomatoes

Lunch: Steak Salad

Dinner: Roasted Salmon Caprese

Day 30

Breakfast: Keto Toast with Chicken and Cucumber

Lunch: Roasted Tofu in Lime Sauce with Green Beans

Dinner: Grilled Pork Tenderloin

Conclusion

There you have it— keto-friendly recipes, which are more than enough get you started in this new journey.

The benefits of the keto diet are countless, and for sure, you'll be delighted at how efficient it is in helping you achieve the ideal weight you've always wanted.

Just make sure that you follow the advice provided in this book, and that you consult your doctor first before getting started.

Good luck!

Lightning Source UK Ltd.
Milton Keynes UK
UKHW050741200123
415680UK00009B/641

9 781953 702647